BAR SOAP FOR BEGINNERS

Easy Recipes, Essential Techniques, Step-By-Step Guide To Crafting Natural Soap For Skin Care And Wellness

ALFORD BARTELL

DISCLAIMER

The author of this book is not linked, associated, authorized, sponsored, or otherwise related to any corporation, business, or person mentioned in this book. This book was written based on the author's expertise, insight, and personal experiences. The material given is intended for educational and informative purposes only and

Table of Contents

CHAPTER ONE 19

Introduction To Bar Soap 19

History And Evolution Of Bar Soap 19

Importance Of Bar Soap In Daily Life 20

Basic Ingredients Used In Bar Soap 22

Benefits Of Using Bar Soap Over Liquid Soap23

Overview Of The Soap-Making Process 25

    1.   Preparing the Ingredients:.................25

    2.   Mixing and Pouring:..........................25

    3.   Curing: 26

CHAPTER TWO 27

Essential Ingredients And Tools 27

Key Ingredients For Soap Making 27

Understanding Oils And Fats..........................28

Lye And Its Role In Soap Making 30

Necessary Equipment And Tools.....................31

Safety Precautions In Handling Ingredients...33

CHAPTER THREE 35

Different Types Of Bar Soap............................35

Handmade Vs. Commercial Bar Soap.............35

Types Of Oils And Their Benefits 37

Fragrances And Essential Oils.....................39

Additives And Natural Colorants....................41

Specialty Soaps...................................43

CHAPTER FOUR...................................47

The Science Of Saponification 47

What Is Saponification? 47

Chemical Reactions Involved........................48

Importance Of Accurate Measurements 50

Temperature Control In Soap Making.............51

Common Mistakes And How To Avoid Them ..53

   1.   Incorrect Measurements: 53

   2.   Improper Temperature Control: 53

   3.   Rushing the Process: 54

   4.   Inadequate Mixing: 54

   5.   Not Wearing Protective Gear:...............55

CHAPTER FIVE 57

Basic Soap Making Methods........................57

Cold Process Soap Making.........................57

   Ingredients and Equipment.......................57

Step-by-Step Procedure 57

Prepare Your Work Area: 57

Measure Ingredients: 58

Mix Lye and Water: 58

Heat Oils: 58

Combine Lye and Oils: 58

Additives: 59

Pour into Molds: 59

Unmold and Cure: 59

Hot Process Soap Making 59

Ingredients and Equipment 59

Step-by-Step Procedure 60

Prepare Your Work Area: 60

Measure Ingredients: 60

Mix Lye and Water: 60

Heat Oils: 60

Combine Lye and Oils: 61

Cook the Soap: 61

Add Additives: 61

Pour into Molds: 61

Unmold and Cure: 61

Melt And Pour Soap Making 62

Ingredients and Equipment 62

Step-by-Step Procedure 62

Cut Soap Base: 63

Melt the Soap Base: 63

Add Additives: 63

Pour into Molds: 63

Let it Set: 63

Rebatching Soap 64

Ingredients and Equipment 64

Step-by-Step Procedure 64

Prepare Your Work Area: 64

Grate the Soap: 64

Add Liquid: 65

Heat the Soap: 65

Add Additives: 65

Pour into Molds: 65

Let it Set: 65

Unmold and Use: 66

Comparison Of Methods 66

Cold Process vs. Hot Process 66

Melt and Pour vs. Rebatching......66

Choosing the Right Method 67

CHAPTER SIX 69

Step-By-Step Cold Process Soap Making......69

Preparing Your Workspace And Materials......69

Measuring And Mixing Ingredients 71

Pouring And Molding The Soap......72

Curing And Cutting The Soap......74

Troubleshooting Common Issues......75

CHAPTER SEVEN 79

Adding Colors And Scents 79

Choosing Natural Colorants 79

Mixing And Adding Colors......80

Selecting And Adding Fragrances......82

Essential Oils Vs. Fragrance Oils 83

Ensuring Even Distribution 85

CHAPTER EIGHT 87

Advanced Soap Making Techniques......87

Swirling And Layering Designs......87

Swirling Designs:......87

Layering Designs:......88

Tips for Success: 88

Embedding Objects In Soap....................89

    Choosing Objects: 89

    Embedding Process: 89

    Safety Considerations: 90

    Finishing Touches: 90

Creating Soap With Exfoliants.................91

    Choosing Exfoliants:..........................91

    Incorporating Exfoliants: 91

    Layering Exfoliants:..........................92

    Benefits and Variations: 92

Using Milk And Other Liquids In Soap 93

    Preparing the Milk: 93

    Adding Lye to Milk:...........................93

    Incorporating Other Liquids:..............94

    Benefits of Milk and Other Liquids:.............94

Techniques For Transparent Soap 95

    Ingredients and Equipment:...............95

    Melting the Soap Base: 95

    Adding Alcohol and Sugar: 96

    Pouring and Setting: 96

Customizing Transparent Soap: 96

Chapter Nine 99

Packaging And Storing Your Soap 99

Proper Curing And Drying 99

Understanding Curing and Drying 99

Steps for Curing 100

1.   Unmolding: 100

2.   Cutting: 100

3.   Curing Racks: 100

4.   Environment: 101

Monitoring Progress 101

Storing Soap For Longevity 101

Optimal Storage Conditions 101

Packaging for Storage 102

Monitoring Stored Soap 102

Creative Packaging Ideas 103

Choosing Packaging Materials 103

Customizing Packaging 103

Practical Packaging Solutions 103

Labeling Requirements And Tips 104

Essential Information 104

Designing Labels 104

Compliance and Regulations 105

Preparing Soap For Gifting Or Selling 105

Gifting Soap 105

Selling Soap 106

Quality Control..106

CHAPTER TEN...107

Troubleshooting And Faqs........................107

Common Soap-Making Problems And Solutions
....107

1. Soap Separating or Curdling: 107

2. Soap Not Setting:...................................108

3. Soap Not Lathering: 108

4. Soap Discoloration:................................108

How To Fix Lye-Heavy Soap 109

1. Testing for Excess Lye: 109

2. Adjusting After the Fact: 110

3. Diluting the Soap:..................................110

4. Preventing Future Issues:......................110

Dealing With Soft Or Crumbly Soap.............111

1. Understanding the Causes: 111

2. Adjusting Recipe and Ratios: 111

3. Proper Curing: 112

4. Rebatching for Fixes: 112

Preventing And Fixing Air Bubbles 112

1. Stirring and Pouring Techniques: 112

2. Using a Stick Blender: 113

3. Troubleshooting Bubbles: 113

4. Ensuring Proper Molding: 113

Frequently Asked Questions From Beginners
....114

CONCLUSION 117

THE END 121

ABOUT THIS BOOK

This book "Bar Soap" delves into the multifaceted world of soap-making, presenting a comprehensive guide for both novice and experienced soap makers. Starting with an introduction to the historical and cultural evolution of bar soap, it highlights the indispensable role that bar soap plays in our daily hygiene routines. The initial chapters underscore the benefits of bar soap over its liquid counterparts, shedding light on its basic ingredients and the overarching process involved in soap making.

Key to understanding soap making is knowledge of the essential ingredients and tools. This book meticulously details the core components such as oils, fats, and lye, emphasizing their roles and the importance of safety when handling these materials.

It also covers the necessary equipment, ensuring that readers are well-prepared to embark on their soap-making journey with confidence.

The variety within bar soaps is extensive, and this book categorizes the differences between handmade and commercial options, the types of oils used, and the benefits of various fragrances and essential oils. It also explores the use of natural colorants and additives and discusses specialty soaps tailored for specific needs like sensitive skin or exfoliation.

"Saponification" is a fundamental concept in soap making, and this book provides a clear explanation of the chemical reactions involved. It stresses the importance of accurate measurements and temperature control, while also offering practical advice on how to avoid common mistakes. This scientific approach is complemented by detailed descriptions of different soap-making methods, including cold process, hot process, melt and pour, and rebatching.

For those interested in the intricacies of soap crafting, this book offers a step-by-step guide to cold-process soap making, from preparing the workspace and measuring ingredients to pouring, molding, curing, and cutting the soap. Troubleshooting tips are included to help readers overcome common issues.

Adding colors and scents to soap is an art form in itself, and this book guides on choosing natural colorants, mixing and adding colors, and selecting fragrances. It differentiates between essential oils and fragrance oils and ensures readers can achieve even distribution of these elements in their soap.

Advanced techniques such as swirling, layering, embedding objects, and using exfoliants are covered, along with methods for incorporating milk and other liquids to create unique and transparent soaps. These techniques enable soap makers to elevate their craft and produce visually appealing and functional soaps.

The final chapters focus on the practical aspects of packaging and storing soap. Proper curing and drying techniques are outlined, along with creative packaging ideas and labeling requirements. This section is particularly useful for those looking to gift or sell their handmade soaps, providing professional tips to enhance presentation and marketability.

Lastly, this book addresses common troubleshooting issues and frequently asked questions, offering solutions to problems like lye-heavy soap, soft or crumbly textures, and air bubbles.

This comprehensive approach ensures that readers have a reliable resource to consult as they refine their soap-making skills.

CHAPTER ONE

Introduction To Bar Soap

History And Evolution Of Bar Soap

The history of bar soap dates back to ancient civilizations, with evidence suggesting its use as far back as 2800 B.C. in Babylon. Early soaps were made from a combination of animal fats and wood ash, which produced a cleaning agent effective for both personal hygiene and washing clothes. The ancient Egyptians also used a similar mixture, recognizing the importance of cleanliness for health and spiritual reasons.

During the middle Ages, soap-making became a craft in Europe, particularly in regions like Spain, Italy, and France. Soap makers began to experiment with different ingredients, such as olive oil, and scents to create more luxurious and effective products. The use of soap became more widespread, though it remained a luxury item for the wealthy.

The Industrial Revolution brought significant advancements to soap production. The invention of chemical processes to produce sodium hydroxide (lye) and the discovery of the properties of glycerin revolutionized the soap-making industry. These advancements made soap more affordable and accessible to the general public. Today, bar soap is a common household item, available in various formulations to cater to different skin types and preferences.

Importance Of Bar Soap In Daily Life

Bar soap plays a crucial role in daily hygiene routines. Its primary function is to cleanse the skin by removing dirt, oil, and impurities, which helps prevent infections and skin conditions.

Regular use of bar soap can help maintain healthy skin by keeping it clean and free from harmful bacteria.

In addition to its cleansing properties, bar soap often contains moisturizing ingredients that help maintain the skin's natural moisture balance. This is especially important for individuals with dry or sensitive skin, as it prevents excessive dryness and irritation. The act of lathering and rinsing with bar soap also promotes relaxation and a sense of well-being, making it an essential part of many people's self-care routines.

Bar soap is also environmentally friendly compared to liquid soap. It typically comes with minimal packaging, reducing plastic waste. Additionally, bar soap tends to last longer than liquid soap, as it is easier to control the amount used per wash. This makes it a cost-effective and sustainable choice for personal hygiene.

Basic Ingredients Used In Bar Soap

The basic ingredients used in bar soap are simple yet effective. The primary components include fats or oils, lye (sodium hydroxide), and water. These ingredients undergo a chemical reaction called saponification, which produces soap and glycerin.

Fats and oils are the core of any soap recipe. Common choices include olive oil, coconut oil, palm oil, and shea butter. Each oil brings different properties to the soap, such as moisturizing, lathering, and hardness. Olive oil, for example, is known for its gentle and moisturizing qualities, while coconut oil provides a rich lather.

Lye is a crucial component in soap making, as it reacts with the fats and oils to create soap. While handling lye requires caution due to its caustic nature, the final product contains no lye, as it is completely consumed in the saponification process.

Water is used to dissolve the lye and mix it with the oils. It also helps to control the consistency of the soap mixture during the saponification process. Optional ingredients like essential oils, colorants, and exfoliates can be added to enhance the soap's fragrance, appearance, and texture.

Benefits Of Using Bar Soap Over Liquid Soap

Bar soap offers several benefits over liquid soap, making it a preferred choice for many. Firstly, bar soap is generally more cost-effective. A single bar lasts longer than an equivalent amount of liquid soap, as it is easier to control the amount used. This makes bar soap a budget-friendly option for households.

Bar soap is also environmentally friendly. It usually comes in minimal packaging, often just a simple paper wrapper or cardboard box, reducing plastic waste significantly. In contrast, liquid soap is typically packaged in plastic bottles, contributing to environmental pollution.

Another advantage of bar soap is its versatility. It can be used for various purposes, including washing hands, body, and even hair in some cases. Many bar soaps are formulated with natural ingredients that are gentle on the skin, making them suitable for individuals with sensitive skin or allergies. Additionally, bar soaps often contain fewer synthetic chemicals and preservatives compared to liquid soaps, making them a healthier choice for your skin.

Overview Of The Soap-Making Process

The soap-making process involves several steps, but it can be simplified into three main stages: preparing the ingredients, mixing and pouring, and curing.

1.   **Preparing the Ingredients:** Start by gathering the necessary ingredients and equipment. You'll need fats or oils, lye, water, and any optional additives like essential oils or colorants. Measure the ingredients accurately to ensure a successful saponification process.

2.   **Mixing and Pouring:** Dissolve the lye in water, following safety precautions to avoid chemical burns. Once the lye solution cools, mix it with the melted fats or oils. Stir the mixture until it reaches "trace," a stage where it thickens and leaves a trail when drizzled on itself.

Add any optional ingredients, then pour the mixture into a mold.

3.   **Curing:** Allow the soap to harden in the mold for 24-48 hours before removing it. Cut the soap into bars and let them cure in a well-ventilated area for 4-6 weeks. This curing process allows the soap to harden and ensures that it is mild and safe to use.

By following these steps, beginners can successfully make their bar soap at home, enjoying the benefits of a personalized, natural cleansing product.

CHAPTER TWO

Essential Ingredients And Tools

Key Ingredients For Soap Making

To make bar soap, you'll need a few essential ingredients that form the basis of the soap-making process. These ingredients include oils, fats, lye, and water. Each component plays a critical role in creating a balanced and effective soap.

Oils and fats are the primary building blocks of soap. Commonly used oils include olive oil, coconut oil, palm oil, and sunflower oil. Each oil has different properties that affect the soap's hardness, lather, and moisturizing qualities. For example, coconut oil is known for its excellent lathering properties, while olive oil provides a creamy lather and is gentle on the skin.

Lye, also known as sodium hydroxide, is a crucial ingredient in soap making. When combined with oils and fats, it triggers a chemical reaction called saponification. This process transforms the oils and lye into soap and glycerin, a natural moisturizer. It's important to use 100% pure lye to ensure the best results.

Water is used to dissolve the lye before it's mixed with the oils. Distilled water is preferred because it's free from impurities that could affect the soap-making process. Tap water may contain minerals and chemicals that can interfere with the reaction between the lye and oils.

Understanding Oils And Fats

Oils and fats are the heart of any bar soap recipe. Each type of oil contributes different characteristics to the final product. Understanding these properties will help you create a soap that meets your specific needs and preferences.

Olive oil is a staple in soap-making due to its skin-conditioning properties. It produces a mild and gentle soap that is suitable for all skin types. However, it creates a softer bar that takes longer to cure.

Coconut oil is valued for its ability to produce a hard, white soap with a fluffy lather. It's often used in combination with other oils to balance its strong cleansing properties, which can be drying if used in excess.

Palm oil is another popular choice, providing a balance between hardness, lather, and conditioning. It's important to source palm oil sustainably to avoid contributing to environmental issues.

Sunflower oil is rich in vitamins A and E, offering nourishing and conditioning benefits. It's usually used in combination with harder oils to improve the soap's moisturizing qualities.

Lye And Its Role In Soap Making

Lye, or sodium hydroxide, is a critical ingredient in the soap-making process. It's responsible for the chemical reaction that transforms oils and fats into soap and glycerin. Without lye, there is no soap – only a mixture of oils and water.

Handling lye requires caution, as it's a caustic substance that can cause burns if it comes into contact with skin. Always wear protective gear, including gloves, goggles, and long sleeves, when working with lye. Ensure you're in a well-ventilated area to avoid inhaling fumes.

When lye is mixed with water, it generates heat. Always add lye to water, not the other way around, to prevent a dangerous reaction. The mixture will become very hot and should be allowed to cool before combining it with oils.

The amount of lye needed depends on the types and amounts of oils used. Soap calculators are available online to help you determine the correct proportions. Accurate measurement is crucial to ensure the soap is properly saponified and safe to use.

Necessary Equipment And Tools

Having the right equipment and tools is essential for successful soap making. These items will help you measure, mix, and mold your ingredients safely and efficiently.

A digital scale is crucial for accurately measuring oils, lye, and water. Precision is key in soap making, and even small deviations can affect the final product.

Mixing bowls made of heat-resistant plastic, stainless steel, or tempered glass are ideal for combining ingredients. Avoid using aluminum or other reactive metals, as they can react with lye.

A stick blender, also known as an immersion blender, helps speed up the saponification process by thoroughly mixing the lye solution with the oils. This tool is preferred over hand stirring, which can take much longer.

Thermometers are necessary to monitor the temperatures of the lye solution and oils before mixing them. Ensuring both are within the same temperature range (around 100-110°F) helps achieve a smooth blend and proper saponification.

Soap molds come in various shapes and sizes, from simple loaf molds to intricate silicone designs. Line molds with parchment paper or use flexible silicone molds for easy removal of the finished soap.

Safety Precautions In Handling Ingredients

Safety is paramount when making soap, especially when working with lye. Following these precautions will help ensure a safe and successful soap-making experience.

Always work in a well-ventilated area or near an open window to avoid inhaling lye fumes. Using a respirator mask can provide additional protection.

Wear protective gear, including long sleeves, gloves, and goggles, to prevent lye from coming into contact with your skin and eyes. Keep a bottle of vinegar nearby to neutralize any accidental lye spills on your skin.

Keep children and pets away from your soap-making area to prevent accidents.

Lye is extremely dangerous if ingested or splashed onto the skin.

Carefully measure all ingredients, especially lye. Use a dedicated set of utensils and containers for soap making, and do not repurpose them for food preparation.

Label all containers and tools used for soap-making to avoid confusion and accidental contamination. Store lye in a secure, dry place away from moisture and out of reach of children and pets.

By understanding the essential ingredients and tools, as well as the necessary safety precautions, you'll be well-prepared to embark on your soap-making journey with confidence.

CHAPTER THREE

Different Types Of Bar Soap

Handmade Vs. Commercial Bar Soap

Handmade bar soap and commercial bar soap differ significantly in their ingredients, production methods, and overall benefits. Handmade soaps are typically crafted in small batches using natural ingredients and traditional methods such as cold process, hot process, or melt and pour. These soaps often contain high-quality oils, butter, and essential oils, providing numerous skin benefits and a luxurious feel. Additionally, handmade soaps usually retain glycerin, a natural byproduct of the soap-making process, which acts as a humectant, drawing moisture into the skin and keeping it hydrated.

In contrast, commercial bar soaps are mass-produced using synthetic detergents, preservatives, and artificial fragrances. These soaps are often stripped of glycerin to increase shelf life, resulting in a product that can be drying to the skin. Commercial soaps are designed for efficiency and cost-effectiveness, often at the expense of quality and skin health. They are typically produced through continuous processes in large manufacturing plants, which allow for consistent and uniform bars but lack the personalized touch of handmade varieties.

For beginners interested in soap making, starting with handmade soap can be a rewarding experience. It allows for creativity in choosing ingredients and personalizing each batch. While commercial soaps offer convenience and availability, handmade soaps provide a unique opportunity to create a customized product tailored to individual skin needs and preferences.

Types Of Oils And Their Benefits

Oils are the backbone of any bar soap, each offering distinct properties that influence the soap's texture, lather, and skin benefits. Common oils used in soap making include olive oil, coconut oil, palm oil, and castor oil, among others.

Olive oil is highly valued for its moisturizing properties and gentle nature, making it suitable for all skin types, especially sensitive or dry skin. It produces a creamy lather and contributes to a hard, long-lasting bar. Coconut oil, on the other hand, is known for its cleansing abilities and ability to produce a rich, bubbly lather. It is excellent for removing dirt and oil but can be drying if used in excess, so it's often balanced with other moisturizing oils.

Palm oil contributes to a hard bar and stable lather, while also being rich in vitamins A and E, which promote skin health. However, ethical and sustainable sourcing of palm oil is crucial due to environmental concerns. Castor oil is a powerful humectant and emollient, drawing moisture to the skin and adding a silky feel to the soap. It also boosts lather, making it a favorite for those who prefer a foamy wash.

Other oils such as avocado oil, sweet almond oil, and jojoba oil can be used to tailor soap recipes to specific skin needs, offering benefits like extra hydration, anti-inflammatory properties, and skin softening. Experimenting with different oils allows soap makers to create unique blends that cater to their preferences and skin types.

Fragrances and essential oils add a sensory experience to bar soaps, making each use enjoyable and therapeutic. Essential oils are derived from plants and carry the aromatic compounds that give them their distinct scents and therapeutic properties. Popular essential oils for soap making include lavender, peppermint, eucalyptus, tea tree, and citrus oils like lemon and orange.

Lavender essential oil is known for its calming and relaxing properties, making it ideal for evening soaps or those aimed at reducing stress. Peppermint oil provides a refreshing and invigorating scent, perfect for morning showers to wake up the senses. Eucalyptus oil has a cooling effect and is often used in soaps intended for respiratory relief or muscle relaxation.

Tea tree oil is celebrated for its antibacterial and antifungal properties, making it suitable for acne-prone skin or soaps designed to cleanse deeply. Citrus oils, such as lemon and orange, offer a bright and uplifting aroma, adding a cheerful note to any soap.

In addition to essential oils, fragrance oils can be used to achieve specific scents not available in nature, such as "ocean breeze" or "pumpkin spice." However, it's important to choose high-quality, skin-safe fragrance oils to avoid irritation.

When incorporating scents into soap, it's crucial to follow recommended usage rates to ensure safety and effectiveness. Too much essential oil can cause skin irritation, while too little might not provide the desired aroma. Beginners should start with tried-and-true recipes and gradually experiment with different combinations to find their perfect scent profile.

Additives And Natural Colorants

Additives and natural colorants enhance the visual appeal and functionality of bar soaps, providing a touch of creativity and additional skin benefits. Common additives include exfoliates, clays, botanicals, and milk, each bringing unique properties to the soap.

Exfoliants like oatmeal, ground coffee, and sea salt add texture and provide gentle scrubbing action, helping to remove dead skin cells and improve circulation. Oatmeal is soothing and suitable for sensitive skin, while coffee grounds can invigorate and energize. Sea salt creates a mineral-rich bar that can help detoxify and balance the skin.

Clays such as kaolin, bentonite, and French green clay add natural color and absorb excess oils, making them ideal for oily or acne-prone skin. Kaolin clay is gentle and can be used in soaps for all skin types, while bentonite clay is more absorbent and suited for deep cleansing.

Botanicals like dried flowers, herbs, and seeds not only add aesthetic appeal but also infuse the soap with their beneficial properties. Lavender buds, rose petals, and chamomile flowers are popular choices, each bringing soothing effects.

Natural colorants such as spirulina, activated charcoal, and turmeric provide vibrant hues without synthetic dyes. Spirulina gives a rich green color and is packed with antioxidants, while activated charcoal creates a striking black bar and is known for its detoxifying properties. Turmeric adds a warm golden color and has anti-inflammatory benefits.

Using these additives and colorants allows soap makers to create visually stunning and beneficial bars that cater to various skin needs and preferences.

Specialty Soaps

Specialty soaps are crafted to address specific skin concerns or provide particular benefits, making them ideal for those with unique needs. Soaps for sensitive skin, exfoliating soaps, and therapeutic soaps are some examples of specialty varieties.

Soaps for sensitive skin are formulated with gentle ingredients to avoid irritation. These soaps often exclude synthetic fragrances and harsh chemicals, opting for mild oils like olive and avocado, and soothing additives such as oatmeal or calendula. Essential oils like chamomile and lavender can be used in minimal amounts to provide a calming scent without causing sensitivity.

Exfoliating soaps contain natural exfoliates that help remove dead skin cells, leaving the skin smooth and refreshed. Ingredients like ground almonds, poppy seeds, or finely ground pumice can be added to create different levels of exfoliation. These soaps are beneficial for rough or dry areas of the body, such as elbows and heels, and can help improve the skin's texture and appearance.

Therapeutic soaps are designed to address specific skin issues or provide relief from conditions like eczema, psoriasis, or acne. Ingredients like neem oil, tea tree oil, and colloidal oatmeal are commonly used for their antibacterial, antifungal, and anti-inflammatory properties.

These soaps aim to soothe and heal troubled skin, providing a gentle yet effective cleansing experience.

Creating specialty soaps involves understanding the unique properties of various ingredients and how they can be combined to achieve the desired effect. By experimenting with different formulations, soap makers can produce bars that cater to a wide range of skin types and concerns.

CHAPTER FOUR

The Science Of Saponification

What Is Saponification?

Saponification is the fundamental chemical process in soap making, where fats or oils react with an alkali, typically sodium hydroxide (lye), to form soap and glycerin. This reaction is essential for transforming the oils and fats into a solid, usable soap that cleans and lathers effectively. Understanding saponification is crucial for any soap maker, as it determines the quality and properties of the final product.

During saponification, triglycerides (the main components of fats and oils) react with lye to produce soap and glycerol (glycerin). The triglycerides break down into their constituent fatty acids and glycerin, which then react with the lye to form soap molecules. This reaction can be summarized by the equation: Fat+Lye→Soap+Glycerintext {Fat} + text {Lye} rightarrow text {Soap} + text {Glycerin} Fat+Lye→Soap+Glycerin

Different oils and fats have varying saponification values, meaning they require different amounts of lye to convert them into soap. This is why accurate measurements are crucial, as using too much or too little lye can affect the soap's properties and safety.

Chemical Reactions Involved

The chemical reaction of saponification involves the hydrolysis of triglycerides. Triglycerides, composed of glycerol and three fatty acids, react with the hydroxide ions from lye.

This process breaks the ester bonds in the triglycerides, releasing glycerol and forming soap molecules.

The reaction can be broken down into two main stages:

Hydrolysis of Triglycerides: The triglycerides are broken down into glycerol and free fatty acids.

Neutralization: The free fatty acids react with the lye to form soap and water.

For instance, when using olive oil (which contains a high percentage of oleic acid), the saponification reaction with sodium hydroxide would look like this:

$$C_3H_5(OOCR)_3 + 3NaOH \rightarrow 3RCOONa + C_3H_5(OH)_3$$

\text{C}_3\text{H}_5(\text{OOCR})_3 + 3\text{NaOH} \rightarrow 3\text{RCOONa} + \text{C}_3\text{H}_5(\text{OH})_3C3H5(OOCR)3+3NaOH→3RCOONa+C3H5(OH)3Here,

C3H5(OOCR)3\text{C}_3\text{H}_5(\text{OOCR})_3C3H5(OOCR)3represents the triglyceride, NaOH\text{NaOH}NaOH is the sodium hydroxide, RCOONa\text{RCOONa}RCOONa is the soap, and C3H5(OH)3\text{C}_3\text{H}_5(\text{OH})_3C3H5(OH)3 is glycerol.

Importance Of Accurate Measurements

Accurate measurements are vital in soap-making to ensure the correct ratio of oils to lye. This balance is necessary to avoid having too much lye (which can make the soap harsh and irritating) or too much oil (which can result in a greasy, unusable product).

Using a lye calculator is a practical approach to achieving precise measurements. These calculators help determine the exact amount of lye needed for a given amount of oil based on their saponification values. For example, if you are using 500 grams of coconut oil, the lye calculator will provide the specific amount of lye required to saponify the oil completely.

Furthermore, measuring ingredients by weight rather than volume ensures consistency and accuracy. A digital scale is a valuable tool in this process, as it allows for precise measurement of both oils and lye. This precision is especially important when scaling recipes up or down.

Temperature Control In Soap Making

Temperature control is a critical aspect of the soap-making process. The temperature at which oils and lye are mixed can significantly impact the saponification process and the final soap quality. Ideally, both the lye solution and the melted oils should be within a specific temperature range, typically between 100°F and 120°F (38°C to 49°C).

Maintaining this temperature range ensures that the saponification reaction proceeds smoothly without causing the soap to "seize" (harden prematurely) or remain too liquid. Using a digital thermometer helps monitor the temperatures accurately. If the temperatures are too high, the soap may harden too quickly, resulting in a crumbly texture. Conversely, if too low, the saponification process may be too slow, leading to incomplete reactions.

To manage temperatures effectively, prepare the lye solution first and allow it to cool while you melt and mix the oils. This approach helps synchronize the temperatures, making it easier to combine them at the right moment. Additionally, working in a controlled environment where sudden temperature changes are minimized can also help maintain consistency.

Common Mistakes And How To Avoid Them

Several common mistakes can occur during soap making, especially for beginners. Recognizing and avoiding these pitfalls can help ensure successful and high-quality soap production.

1.   **Incorrect Measurements:** One of the most frequent mistakes is inaccurate measurements of oils and lye. Always use a digital scale to measure ingredients by weight and double-check calculations using a lye calculator. Even a small deviation can significantly impact the soap's quality and safety.

2.   **Improper Temperature Control:** Mixing oils and lye at incorrect temperatures can cause various issues, such as soap seizing or incomplete

saponification. Always monitor and maintain the temperature of both components within the recommended range (100°F to 120°F). Use a digital thermometer for precise readings.

3.   **Rushing the Process:** Patience is key in soap making. Allow the lye solution to cool appropriately and give the soap mixture enough time to reach trace (the stage where the mixture thickens and leaves trails on the surface). Rushing these steps can lead to incomplete mixing or uneven texture.

4.   **Inadequate Mixing:** Failing to mix the soap batter thoroughly can result in uneven saponification, leading to pockets of unreacted lye or oil. Use a stick blender to blend the mixture until it reaches a uniform trace. Ensure all ingredients are evenly incorporated.

5.   **Not Wearing Protective Gear:** Handling lye requires proper safety precautions. Always wear gloves, goggles, and long sleeves to protect your skin and eyes from potential splashes. Work in a well-ventilated area to avoid inhaling fumes.

By being aware of these common mistakes and taking the necessary precautions, you can produce high-quality, safe, and effective soap. Practice, attention to detail, and following best practices will enhance your soap-making skills over time.

CHAPTER FIVE

Basic Soap Making Methods

Cold Process Soap Making

Ingredients and Equipment

To begin the cold process of soap making, gather your ingredients and equipment. You'll need oils (such as olive oil, coconut oil, and palm oil), lye (sodium hydroxide), water, essential oils, and any desired colorants. Equipment includes a digital scale, safety goggles, gloves, a stick blender, soap molds, and a thermometer.

Step-by-Step Procedure

Prepare Your Work Area: Ensure your work area is well-ventilated. Lay out all your materials and equipment. Put on your safety goggles and gloves to protect yourself from the lye.

Measure Ingredients: Accurately measure your oils and lye using the digital scale. It's crucial to get precise measurements to ensure the chemical reaction occurs correctly.

Mix Lye and Water: Slowly add the lye to the water (never the other way around) and stir until the lye is fully dissolved. This mixture will heat up quickly and emit fumes, so do this in a well-ventilated area and let it cool.

Heat Oils: While the lye solution cools, heat your oils in a pot until they reach about 100-120°F (38-49°C). Use the thermometer to check the temperature.

Combine Lye and Oils: When both the lye solution and oils are at the same temperature range, carefully pour the lye solution into the oils. Use the stick blender to mix until you reach "trace"—when the mixture thickens and leaves a trail on the surface.

Additives: Add essential oils, colorants, or other additives at trace. Blend them in thoroughly.

Pour into Molds: Pour the soap mixture into your molds, smooth the top with a spatula, and cover with a towel to retain heat. Let it sit for 24-48 hours to harden.

Unmold and Cure: After the soap has hardened, remove it from the molds and cut it into bars if necessary. Let the soap bars cure in a well-ventilated area for 4-6 weeks. This curing time allows the soap to fully saponify and become milder.

Hot Process Soap Making

Ingredients and Equipment

The ingredients for hot process soap making are similar to cold process soap making: oils, lye, water, essential oils, and colorants. You'll also need a digital scale, safety goggles, gloves, a slow cooker (Crock-Pot), a stick blender, soap molds, and a thermometer.

Step-by-Step Procedure

Prepare Your Work Area: Set up your workspace with all your materials and equipment. Wear safety goggles and gloves for protection.

Measure Ingredients: Weigh your oils and lye accurately using the digital scale.

Mix Lye and Water: Add the lye to the water slowly and stir until fully dissolved. This mixture will heat up and emit fumes, so work in a well-ventilated area and let it cool.

Heat Oils: Place the oils in the slow cooker and heat until melted and mixed.

Combine Lye and Oils: When the lye solution and oils are at the right temperature, carefully add the lye solution to the oils. Use the stick blender to mix until you reach a trace.

Cook the Soap: Cover the slow cooker and cook the soap mixture on low heat. Stir occasionally. The soap will go through different phases: it will become translucent and then turn into a gel-like consistency. This process usually takes 1-2 hours.

Add Additives: Once the soap reaches the gel phase, add your essential oils, colorants, or other additives. Stir them in well.

Pour into Molds: Pour the soap mixture into your molds and smooth the top with a spatula. Let it sit until it hardens, usually 24 hours.

Unmold and Cure: After the soap has hardened, remove it from the molds and cut it into bars if necessary. While hot process soap can be used immediately, it's best to let it cure for a week or two to allow excess moisture to evaporate and improve the soap's hardness.

Melt And Pour Soap Making

Ingredients and Equipment

For melt-and-pour soap making, you need a pre-made soap base, which can be purchased online or at craft stores. Additional ingredients include essential oils, colorants, and other additives. Equipment includes a microwave-safe container, soap molds, and a stirring utensil.

Step-by-Step Procedure

Prepare Your Work Area: Lay out all your materials and equipment. This method doesn't involve lye, so safety gear isn't necessary, but it's still good to have a clean and organized workspace.

Cut Soap Base: Cut the soap base into small, even pieces to ensure they melt uniformly.

Melt the Soap Base: Place the soap base pieces in a microwave-safe container and heat in the microwave in short bursts (20-30 seconds), stirring in between, until fully melted. Alternatively, you can use a double boiler on the stove.

Add Additives: Once the soap base is melted, add your essential oils, colorants, and any other additives. Stir well to distribute evenly.

Pour into Molds: Pour the melted soap base into your soap molds. Tap the molds gently to release any air bubbles.

Let it Set: Allow the soap to cool and harden completely. This usually takes a few hours.

Unmold and Use: Once the soap is fully hardened, remove it from the molds. Melt and pour soap can be used immediately, as it doesn't require curing.

Rebatching Soap

Ingredients and Equipment

For rebatching soap, you'll need previously made cold process or hot process soap that has cured, a grater, a pot or slow cooker, water or milk, a digital scale, soap molds, and a stirring utensil.

Step-by-Step Procedure

Prepare Your Work Area: Set up your workspace with all your materials and equipment.

Grate the Soap: Grate your cured soap bars into small, fine pieces. The finer the soap pieces, the faster they will melt.

Add Liquid: Weigh the grated soap and add a small amount of water or milk (about 1 ounce of liquid per pound of soap). This will help the soap melt and become pliable.

Heat the Soap: Place the grated soap and liquid in a pot or slow cooker. Heat gently over low heat, stirring occasionally, until the soap melts and forms a thick, lumpy paste. This can take several hours.

Add Additives: Once the soap has melted into a paste, you can add essential oils, colorants, or other additives. Stir well to incorporate.

Pour into Molds: Spoon the soap paste into your molds, pressing down to eliminate air pockets. Smooth the top with a spatula.

Let it Set: Allow the soap to cool and harden completely. This can take 24-48 hours.

Unmold and Use: Once the soap is fully hardened, remove it from the molds. Rebatched soap doesn't require additional curing and can be used immediately.

Comparison Of Methods

Cold Process vs. Hot Process

Cold-process soap making is ideal for those who enjoy a hands-on, scientific approach and appreciate the artistic freedom of creating intricate designs and patterns. However, it requires patience due to the long curing time. Hot process soap making, on the other hand, allows for quicker use of the soap, as it can be used almost immediately after making, though it lacks the smooth finish and intricate design potential of cold process soaps.

Melt and Pour vs. Rebatching

Melt-and-pour soap making is the easiest and fastest method, making it perfect for beginners or those short on time. It eliminates the need for handling lye and allows for immediate use of the soap. Rebatching is great for recycling and reusing old soap, but it can be more time-consuming and result in a rustic appearance.

Choosing the Right Method

The choice of method depends on your personal preferences, time constraints, and comfort level with handling lye. Cold process and hot process methods provide more control over the ingredients and customization, while melt and pour and rebatching are more straightforward and beginner-friendly. Each method has its unique advantages, allowing you to choose the one that best fits your needs and resources.

CHAPTER SIX

Step-By-Step Cold Process Soap Making

Preparing Your Workspace And Materials

When preparing your workspace for cold-process soap making, it's essential to ensure that your environment is clean, organized, and safe. Begin by clearing a dedicated area in your kitchen or a well-ventilated room. Cover your work surface with newspapers or a plastic sheet to protect it from spills and stains. Gather all the materials and equipment you'll need, including oils, lye (sodium hydroxide), distilled water, essential oils, and any colorants or additives.

Safety is paramount in soap making. Always wear protective gear, including gloves, goggles, and long sleeves, to protect your skin and eyes from the caustic nature of lye. Ensure you have access to a sink or a source of running water in case of accidental spills. Keep vinegar nearby to neutralize any lye that might come into contact with your skin.

Organize your tools and equipment. You'll need a digital scale for accurate measurements, heat-resistant containers for mixing lye and oils, a stainless steel or heat-resistant plastic spoon for stirring, and silicone molds for shaping your soap. Additionally, have a thermometer to monitor temperatures, a stick blender for emulsifying the mixture, and paper towels or cloths for cleaning up spills. By having everything in place, you'll create a smooth and efficient soap-making process.

Measuring And Mixing Ingredients

Accurate measurement of ingredients is crucial in cold-process soap making. Start by weighing your oils using a digital scale. Common oils used include olive oil, coconut oil, palm oil, and castor oil. Each oil contributes different properties to the soap, such as lather, hardness, and moisturizing qualities. Combine your oils in a heat-resistant container and gently heat them to the recommended temperature, typically around 100-110°F (38-43°C).

Next, measure the lye and distilled water separately. Slowly add the lye to the water, never the other way around, to prevent dangerous reactions. Stir the mixture gently until the lye is fully dissolved. The lye solution will become very hot, so let it cool down to the same temperature range as the oils.

Use a thermometer to ensure both the oil and lye solutions are within 5°F (2-3°C) of each other before mixing.

Once the oils and lye solution are at the correct temperatures, slowly pour the lye solution into the oils. Use a stick blender to mix the ingredients, pulsing and stirring intermittently to avoid air bubbles. Continue blending until you reach "trace," a stage where the mixture thickens and leaves a trail when drizzled on the surface. This usually takes a few minutes and indicates that the oils and lye have emulsified, forming the soap base.

Pouring And Molding The Soap

After achieving trace, it's time to add any desired colorants, fragrances, or additives to your soap mixture. Be sure to mix them thoroughly to ensure even distribution.

Pour the soap batter into your prepared molds, using a spatula to scrape every last bit from the container. Gently tap the molds on the counter to release any trapped air bubbles and smooth the surface of the soap.

Cover the molds with a piece of cardboard or plastic wrap and insulate them with a towel or blanket. This helps to maintain a consistent temperature, promoting the saponification process. Leave the soap undisturbed for 24 to 48 hours, during which it will harden and complete the initial curing phase.

Once the soap has hardened, carefully unmold it. If the soap is difficult to remove, place the mold in the freezer for 30 minutes to help release it. Cut the soap into bars using a soap cutter or a sharp knife. The size and shape of the bars can be customized to your preference.

Handle the freshly cut soap with care, as it will still be caustic and soft at this stage.

Curing And Cutting The Soap

Curing is a crucial step in cold process soap making, as it allows the soap to fully harden and milden over time. Arrange the freshly cut soap bars on a drying rack or a piece of wax paper, ensuring that they are spaced apart to allow air circulation. Place the rack in a cool, dry, and well-ventilated area, away from direct sunlight and humidity.

The curing process typically takes 4 to 6 weeks, during which the soap undergoes saponification and loses excess moisture. This results in a harder, longer-lasting bar with a gentler pH. Turn the bars occasionally to ensure even curing and prevent any warping or uneven drying.

While curing, check the soap periodically for any signs of issues, such as mold or discoloration. If you notice any problems, address them promptly by trimming affected areas or discarding compromised bars. Once the curing period is complete, the soap is ready for use. Store the cured soap in a cool, dry place, ideally wrapped in paper or placed in a breathable container to maintain its quality.

Troubleshooting Common Issues

Cold process soap making can sometimes present challenges, even for experienced soap makers. One common issue is "seizing," where the soap mixture thickens too quickly, making it difficult to pour into molds. This can be caused by fragrance oils with high alcohol content or mixing at too high a temperature. To prevent seizing, choose fragrance oils specifically designed for cold-process soap and ensure your oil and lye solutions are within the recommended temperature range.

Another common problem is soap that remains soft or sticky after the initial curing period. This can result from using too much liquid in the recipe or not allowing sufficient curing time. Ensure you follow the recipe measurements accurately and give your soap enough time to cure fully. If the soap remains soft, extend the curing period by a few more weeks.

Air bubbles or pockets in the soap can occur if the mixture is not properly tapped or stirred before pouring. To avoid this, gently tap your molds on the counter to release trapped air and stir the mixture thoroughly before pouring. If you still encounter air pockets, you can use a needle or toothpick to pop them while the soap is still soft.

By understanding these common issues and their solutions, you can improve your soap-making skills and create high-quality, beautiful bars of soap with confidence.

CHAPTER SEVEN

Adding Colors And Scents

Choosing Natural Colorants

When it comes to adding colors to your homemade bar soap, natural colorants are a fantastic option. These colorants are derived from natural sources like plants, minerals, and clays, ensuring that your soap is free from synthetic dyes and chemicals. Some popular natural colorants include spirulina (for green), turmeric (for yellow), activated charcoal (for black), and cocoa powder (for brown).

To incorporate these into your soap, you need to prepare them properly. For powders like spirulina and turmeric, it's essential to mix them with a small amount of oil or water before adding them to your soap mixture. This helps to prevent clumping and ensures an even distribution of color throughout your soap. Clays, such as kaolin or bentonite, should be mixed with water to form a smooth paste before being added to your soap base.

Experimenting with different natural colorants can be fun and rewarding. Each batch of soap can take on a unique appearance depending on the amount and type of colorant used. Remember to start with small amounts and gradually increase until you achieve the desired hue, as some natural colorants can be quite potent.

Mixing And Adding Colors

Once you have chosen your colorants and prepared them accordingly, the next step is to mix and add them to your soap base. It's crucial to add the colorants at the right stage of the soap-making process to ensure an even and vibrant color throughout your bars. Typically, you will add colorants after the soap base has melted but before it starts to thicken or set.

Begin by melting your soap base using a double boiler or microwave. Once melted, remove it from the heat source and allow it to cool slightly. Gradually add your prepared colorant, stirring continuously to ensure it disperses evenly. Use a whisk or stick blender for thorough mixing, especially if you're working with larger batches.

To achieve multiple colors in one soap bar, you can divide your soap base into separate containers, each with a different colorant. Pour these colored bases into your mold in layers or swirls to create beautiful, multi-colored designs. If you're making layered soap, allow each layer to set slightly before pouring the next to prevent the colors from blending too much.

Adding fragrance to your soap is where you can get creative and personalize each batch. Fragrances can evoke different moods and experiences, making your soap not only a cleansing tool but also a sensory delight. When selecting fragrances, consider who will be using the soap and what types of scents they might enjoy. Popular choices include lavender, citrus, peppermint, and eucalyptus.

Fragrances can come from either essential oils or fragrance oils. Essential oils are natural extracts from plants, offering not only pleasant aromas but also various therapeutic benefits. Fragrance oils, on the other hand, are synthetically produced and can offer a wider range of scents, including those that are difficult to find in nature.

When adding your chosen fragrance, measure it carefully according to the recommended usage rates, which are typically provided by the supplier. Overuse of fragrance can lead to skin irritation, so it's essential to follow these guidelines closely. Add the fragrance oil or essential oil to the melted soap base and stir thoroughly to ensure an even distribution of scent.

Essential Oils Vs. Fragrance Oils

Understanding the difference between essential oils and fragrance oils is crucial for making informed decisions about your soap. Essential oils are natural and extracted from various parts of plants, such as flowers, leaves, and roots. They are often preferred for their natural properties and potential therapeutic benefits. However, they can be more expensive and may have limitations in scent variety.

Fragrance oils are synthetic and designed to mimic natural scents or create entirely new aromas. They are generally more affordable and offer a broader range of scents, including those that cannot be derived from nature, such as "ocean breeze" or "cotton candy." While they lack the therapeutic properties of essential oils, they are a practical choice for achieving specific scents in soap making.

When deciding which to use, consider the purpose of your soap. If you aim for a natural, therapeutic product, essential oils are the way to go. For more complex or unique scents, fragrance oils might be better. Always test your chosen oil in a small batch to ensure it behaves well in the soap and does not cause any adverse reactions.

Ensuring Even Distribution

Ensuring the even distribution of colors and scents in your soap is vital for consistency and quality. To achieve this, meticulous mixing is required. After adding your colorants and fragrances, stir the soap base continuously and thoroughly. Use a stick blender or whisk to incorporate all ingredients evenly. This helps to prevent any clumps of color or pockets of fragrance that could cause issues later on.

For layered or swirled soaps, pour slowly and carefully to control the distribution of colors and scents. If you're adding additional ingredients like dried herbs or exfoliates, sprinkle them evenly over the surface before stirring them in gently. This helps to distribute them uniformly throughout the soap.

Finally, once your soap is poured into the mold, tap the mold gently on a flat surface to release any trapped air bubbles. This also helps the ingredients settle evenly. Allow the soap to cool and harden completely before removing it from the mold and cutting it into bars. Proper curing time will ensure the scents and colors remain vibrant and consistent throughout each bar.

CHAPTER EIGHT

Advanced Soap Making Techniques

Swirling And Layering Designs

Swirling and layering designs in soap-making add an artistic flair to your homemade creations. These techniques are popular among experienced soap makers, but with some practice, beginners can also achieve beautiful results.

Swirling Designs: To create a swirl design, you will need multiple colors of soap batter. Divide your soap mixture into separate containers and add different colors to each. Using a stick blender, ensure each color is evenly mixed. Pour the colored soap batters into your mold in a random pattern. To create the swirl effect, use a swirling tool or a simple chopstick to draw intricate patterns through the soap batter.

Move the tool in various directions to create unique designs. Allow the soap to set for 24-48 hours before unmolding and cutting it into bars.

Layering Designs: Layering involves pouring different layers of soap batter one on top of the other. To achieve distinct layers, pour one color of soap into the mold and allow it to set slightly before adding the next layer. This ensures that the layers do not mix. Repeat this process until the mold is filled. You can use a spoon or spatula to create textured layers, adding another dimension to your soap. After pouring all the layers, let the soap harden for 24-48 hours before cutting.

Tips for Success: When creating swirls and layers, ensure that your soap batter is at the right consistency—not too thick or too thin. Use vibrant colors and experiment with different patterns to find your favorite designs.

Patience is key; allow each layer to set slightly to avoid blending.

Embedding Objects In Soap

Embedding objects in soap is a fun and creative way to make your soap unique. You can embed toys, herbs, dried flowers, or even small pieces of soap into your bars.

Choosing Objects: Select objects that are safe for skin contact and will not deteriorate in soap. Popular choices include small plastic toys, dried lavender buds, or pieces of colored soap. Ensure the objects are clean and dry before embedding them.

Embedding Process: Begin by preparing your soap batter as usual. Pour a layer of soap into your mold and allow it to set slightly, but not completely.

Place your chosen objects on the surface of the soap, pressing them in gently. Pour another layer of soap over the objects to cover them. If you want the objects to be visible on the surface, you can embed them after pouring all the soap batter.

Safety Considerations: Make sure that the objects you embed are not sharp or harmful when the soap is used. Avoid using objects that can cause injury or irritation. Test your soap to ensure that the embedded items remain secure and do not fall out during use.

Finishing Touches: Allow the soap to cure for 24-48 hours before unmolding and cutting. The embedded objects will create interesting textures and visuals, making your soap bars stand out. These soaps make great gifts, especially for children when toys are embedded.

Creating Soap With Exfoliants

Adding exfoliates to your soap not only enhances its texture but also provides added skincare benefits. Exfoliants help remove dead skin cells, leaving the skin feeling smooth and refreshed.

Choosing Exfoliants: There are many natural exfoliates to choose from, including oatmeal, coffee grounds, poppy seeds, and ground almonds. Select exfoliates that suit your skin type and desired level of exfoliation. For gentle exfoliation, use finely ground ingredients; for a more intense scrub, use coarser materials.

Incorporating Exfoliants: Prepare your soap batter as usual, but before pouring it into the mold, add your chosen exfoliates. Stir the exfoliates into the soap batter thoroughly to ensure they are evenly distributed. The amount of exfoliate you add depends on your preference, but a general guideline is to use one tablespoon per pound of soap.

Layering Exfoliants: You can create visually appealing soaps by layering different exfoliate. For example, pour a layer of soap batter with coffee grounds, let it set slightly, and then pour another layer with oatmeal. This creates a layered look with varied textures.

Benefits and Variations: Exfoliating soaps are great for areas of the body that need extra attention, like elbows and feet. You can also combine exfoliate with other additives, such as essential oils and butter, to create a luxurious spa-like experience. Experiment with different combinations to find your favorite exfoliating soap recipe.

Using Milk And Other Liquids In Soap

Using milk and other liquids in soap-making adds moisturizing properties and a creamy texture to your soap. Commonly used liquids include cow's milk, goat's milk, coconut milk, and even herbal teas.

Preparing the Milk: Before adding milk to your soap, freeze it in ice cube trays. This helps prevent the milk from scorching when you add lye. Measure the required amount of milk according to your recipe and freeze it in advance.

Adding Lye to Milk: When the milk is frozen, slowly add the lye to the milk cubes, stirring constantly. This process takes longer than adding lye to water, but it prevents the milk from burning and turning brown. The mixture will gradually melt and become a creamy liquid.

Make sure to wear protective gear as you would with any lye solution.

Incorporating Other Liquids: Herbal teas and other liquids can be used in place of water in your soap recipe. Brew a strong tea and let it cool completely before using it as your liquid. Follow the same process as with milk, adding the lye slowly to the cooled tea.

Benefits of Milk and Other Liquids: Milk soaps are highly moisturizing and gentle on the skin, making them ideal for sensitive skin types. Herbal teas can add subtle fragrances and beneficial properties to your soap, depending on the herbs used. Experiment with different liquids to create a range of nourishing soaps.

Techniques For Transparent Soap

Creating transparent soap, also known as glycerin soap, involves a different process than traditional cold or hot process soap making. Transparent soap has a clear appearance and allows light to pass through, making it visually appealing.

Ingredients and Equipment: To make transparent soap, you will need a glycerin soap base, alcohol (such as vodka), sugar, and water. Additionally, you'll need a double boiler or microwave-safe container for melting the soap base, as well as molds for shaping the soap.

Melting the Soap Base: Cut the glycerin soap base into small cubes and melt it using a double boiler or microwave. If using a microwave, heat in short intervals and stir frequently to avoid overheating. Once melted, the soap base should be clear and free of lumps.

Adding Alcohol and Sugar: Dissolve sugar in a small amount of water and add it to the melted soap base. Stir thoroughly to ensure the sugar is completely dissolved. Next, add alcohol to the mixture, which helps make the soap transparent. The ratio of alcohol to soap base should be about 1:3. Stir the mixture until it is well combined and smooth.

Pouring and Setting: Pour the liquid soap into molds and let it cool and harden. This process usually takes several hours. Once the soap has fully set, remove it from the molds. The resulting soap should be clear and ready for use.

Customizing Transparent Soap: You can add colors, fragrances, and other additives to your transparent soap base.

Mica powders and liquid dyes work well for coloring transparent soap, while essential oils can add pleasant scents. Experiment with different combinations to create unique and beautiful soap bars.

By following these advanced soap-making techniques, you can create stunning and unique soap bars that stand out from the crowd. Whether you are swirling colors, embedding objects, adding exfoliate, using milk, or making transparent soap, each method offers endless possibilities for creativity and customization.

CHAPTER NINE

Packaging And Storing Your Soap

Proper Curing And Drying

Understanding Curing and Drying

Curing and drying are essential steps in soap-making that ensure your bars are fully matured, stable, and ready for use. After you have poured your soap into molds, it needs to undergo a curing process. This involves allowing the soap to air dry and harden over some time, typically 4 to 6 weeks. This process helps to complete the saponification reaction, where the fats and lye fully react to form soap, and it also ensures excess water evaporates, resulting in a firmer, longer-lasting bar.

Steps for Curing

1.   **Unmolding:** Once your soap has set and hardened enough to hold its shape (usually 24 to 48 hours), carefully remove it from the mold. The soap should be firm but still a bit soft, as it will harden further during curing.

2.   **Cutting:** If you use a large mold, cut the soap into individual bars using a sharp knife or soap cutter. This helps increase airflow around each bar, which is crucial for even curing.

3.   **Curing Racks:** Place the cut bars on a curing rack or a shelf lined with parchment paper. Ensure that the bars are spaced apart to allow for good air circulation on all sides. Avoid stacking the bars directly on top of each other, as this can lead to uneven curing and potential sticking.

4.   **Environment:** Keep the curing soap in a cool, dry place away from direct sunlight. Excessive heat or moisture can affect the soap's quality and curing process.

Monitoring Progress

During the curing period, periodically check the soap for any signs of issues like sweating or mold. Proper ventilation is key; if your curing area is humid, consider using a dehumidifier or a fan to improve air circulation. The soap will gradually harden and lose moisture, resulting in a harder, more durable bar.

Storing Soap For Longevity

Optimal Storage Conditions

Once your soap is fully cured, proper storage is crucial to maintaining its quality and extending its shelf life. Store your soap in a cool, dry place to prevent it from becoming too soft or developing mold. Ideally, the storage area should be well-ventilated and free from excessive humidity.

Packaging for Storage

For long-term storage, wrap your soap in breathable materials such as wax paper, parchment paper, or a cotton cloth. Avoid plastic wrap, as it traps moisture and can lead to a sticky surface or mold growth. You can also use cardboard boxes or paper bags to protect your soap while allowing it to breathe.

Monitoring Stored Soap

Check stored soap periodically for any signs of deterioration. If the soap appears dry or cracked, it may have been exposed to too much air. Conversely, if it feels sticky or has an unpleasant odor, it may have been exposed to moisture. Proper storage conditions will help preserve the soap's fragrance, texture, and effectiveness.

Creative Packaging Ideas

Choosing Packaging Materials

When it comes to packaging your soap, creativity can enhance both its appeal and functionality. Consider using natural materials such as kraft paper, jute, or burlap for a rustic, eco-friendly look. For a more polished appearance, you can use decorative boxes, tins, or even glass jars.

Customizing Packaging

Personalize your soap packaging to make it stand out. You can use stamps, stickers, or custom labels to add your brand's logo or design. Adding a ribbon or a small charm can also give your soap a unique touch. Ensure that the packaging reflects the quality and care that went into making the soap.

Practical Packaging Solutions

Consider the practicality of your packaging. For instance, if you're packaging soap for gifts or sale, choose materials that protect the soap from damage and maintain its freshness. For bulk packaging, consider using shrink wrap or cellophane bags, which are easy to handle and keep the soap clean.

Labeling Requirements And Tips

Essential Information

Proper labeling is essential for both compliance and customer satisfaction. Each soap label should include the product name, ingredients list, weight or volume, and contact information. If the soap is handmade, it's also useful to include a "handmade" label to highlight its artisanal quality.

Designing Labels

Create labels that are both informative and visually appealing. Use clear, readable fonts and high-quality printing to ensure that the information is legible.

Consider including a brief description of the soap's benefits or any unique features, such as organic ingredients or essential oils.

Compliance and Regulations

Check local regulations regarding labeling requirements for cosmetic products. Some regions may have specific rules about ingredient disclosures, allergen warnings, or claims that can be made. Ensuring your labels comply with these regulations will help you avoid potential legal issues and build trust with your customers.

Preparing Soap For Gifting Or Selling

Gifting Soap

When preparing soap as a gift, presentation is key. Wrap the soap in decorative paper or place it in a gift box with a personalized note. You can also include a small information card about the soap's ingredients and benefits to add a personal touch. Ensure that the packaging is both attractive and functional, protecting the soap during transit.

Selling Soap

For selling soap, focus on both presentation and practicality. Use professional-looking packaging that reflects your brand and appeals to your target market. Ensure the soap is well-protected during shipping and handling. If selling online, consider including high-quality images and detailed product descriptions on your website or marketplace listings.

Quality Control

Before gifting or selling your soap, inspect each bar for any defects or inconsistencies. Ensure that the soap is fully cured and has a uniform appearance. For a professional finish, ensure that all labels and packaging are applied correctly and that the final product meets your quality standards.

CHAPTER TEN

Troubleshooting And Faqs

Common Soap-Making Problems And Solutions

Soap-making can be a fulfilling hobby, but even seasoned crafters can run into issues. Understanding common problems and their solutions will help you refine your process and create consistent, high-quality bars. Here's a breakdown of typical soap-making problems and straightforward solutions to resolve them.

1. Soap Separating or Curdling: This issue often arises due to incorrect temperatures or excessive mixing. To avoid this, ensure that both your lye solution and oils are at the recommended temperatures before combining them.

Mixing should be done until just reaching a light trace—when the mixture thickens but before it becomes too thick to pour.

2. Soap Not Setting: If your soap isn't setting, it might be due to insufficient curing time or improper formulation. Make sure your recipe is balanced and use a reliable lye calculator to verify the ratios. Allow the soap to cure in a cool, dry place for the recommended time, typically 4-6 weeks, to ensure it hardens properly.

3. Soap Not Lathering: Low lather can result from using the wrong type of oils or incorrect saponification. Use oils with high lathering properties, like coconut oil, and check that your lye measurement is accurate. Conduct a test batch to fine-tune your recipe.

4. Soap Discoloration: Discoloration can occur due to the type of oils used or from the addition of certain ingredients like vanilla or citrus. Use antioxidants like Vitamin E to help preserve color and avoid using oils or additives that are prone to discoloring.

How To Fix Lye-Heavy Soap

Lye-heavy soap is a result of using too much lye in your recipe. This condition can lead to a harsh, caustic bar that can be irritating to the skin. Here's how to address and correct this problem:

1. Testing for Excess Lye: First, test your soap with a pH strip. If the pH is higher than 10, it indicates excess lye. If you're still in the initial stages and the soap hasn't fully set, you can remelt and adjust the formulation by adding more fats.

2. Adjusting After the Fact: For already hardened soap, you can try to rebatch it. Grate the soap into small pieces and reheat it in a double boiler with a small amount of distilled water or additional fats (like olive oil). Stir well until it reaches a smooth consistency and pour it into a mold.

3. Diluting the Soap: Another method is to dilute the lye-heavy soap to make it milder. Dissolve the soap in water to create a liquid soap base, then rebatch it or use it as a liquid soap, ensuring it is well-cured before use.

4. Preventing Future Issues: Always use a reliable lye calculator to double-check your ratios before making soap. Invest in quality scales and measuring tools to ensure accuracy.

Dealing With Soft Or Crumbly Soap

Soft or crumbly soap can be frustrating, especially if you've put in the effort to craft a perfect batch. Here's how to address and prevent this issue:

1. Understanding the Causes: Soft soap is usually due to excess water or oils that haven't been fully saponified. Crumbly soap often results from a high percentage of hard oils like palm or coconut that haven't been balanced with soft oils.

2. Adjusting Recipe and Ratios: To fix soft soap, reduce the amount of water used in your recipe or ensure that your soap has had sufficient time to cure. For crumbly soap, balance your recipe with a mix of hard and soft oils to ensure proper consistency.

3. Proper Curing: Ensure your soap is cured in a well-ventilated area. A good cure time for most soap is 4-6 weeks, but some recipes may require more time. Check your soap periodically and ensure it is stored in a cool, dry place.

4. Rebatching for Fixes: If your soap is already made and is too soft or crumbly, consider rebatching it. Grate the soap into small pieces, reheat with a bit of water or additional oils in a double boiler, and stir until the texture improves.

Preventing And Fixing Air Bubbles

Air bubbles can mar the surface of your soap and affect its appearance. Here's how to prevent and fix them:

1. Stirring and Pouring Techniques: To prevent air bubbles, avoid excessive mixing or stirring, which can incorporate air.

Pour your soap batter gently into the mold to minimize bubble formation. Tapping the mold on the counter can help release trapped air.

2. Using a Stick Blender: When blending your soap batter, use a stick blender at a low speed. This helps avoid incorporating too much air. Blend just until you reach a trace and avoid overmixing.

3. Troubleshooting Bubbles: If bubbles appear on the surface after pouring, use a heat gun or blow dryer on a low setting to gently pop them. This technique works well for surface bubbles but be cautious not to overheat the soap.

4. Ensuring Proper Molding: Choose a mold with a smooth interior and avoid overfilling. If you use silicone molds, they are generally better at reducing bubbles due to their flexible nature.

Frequently Asked Questions From Beginners

1. How long should I wait before using my soap?

Most soaps need to be cured for about 4-6 weeks before they're ready to use. This curing time allows the soap to harden and for the saponification process to complete, resulting in a milder, longer-lasting bar.

2. Can I use regular kitchen utensils for soap making?

It's best to use dedicated utensils for soap making. Lye can be corrosive, so avoid using your regular kitchen tools. Invest in heat-resistant bowls, measuring spoons, and spatulas specifically for soap making.

3. What should I do if my soap has an unusual odor?

Unusual odors can result from incorrect curing or the use of incompatible ingredients. Ensure your soap is fully cured in a well-ventilated area and check your recipe for any potential sources of odor. Essential oils can be added to mask or enhance scents.

4. Is it necessary to use a soap mold?

While a soap mold is highly recommended for shaping your bars, you can improvise with household items like silicone baking molds or even plastic containers. Just ensure they are well-lined and suitable for the soap's temperature during curing.

5. Can I modify a soap recipe?

Yes, you can modify soap recipes, but it requires careful adjustments to maintain balance in the lye-to-oil ratio. Use a reliable soap calculator and test new recipes in small batches to ensure proper results.

CONCLUSION

Bar soap, a staple in personal hygiene for centuries remains a timeless choice despite the proliferation of liquid soaps and other cleansing products. Its continued popularity can be attributed to several enduring benefits that make it a preferred option for many individuals.

Firstly, bar soap is celebrated for its simplicity and effectiveness. Unlike liquid soaps, which often require plastic packaging, bar soap comes with minimal environmental impact. This eco-friendly aspect appeals to the growing number of environmentally conscious consumers who seek to reduce their carbon footprint. Additionally, the lack of water in bar soap means that users can enjoy a more concentrated formula, which often results in longer-lasting use and less product wastage.

Moreover, bar soap is highly versatile and can cater to various skin types and needs. From moisturizing bars enriched with essential oils to exfoliating bars with natural scrubs, the variety available allows consumers to choose products tailored to their specific skin concerns. This versatility extends to its use in different settings, such as home bathrooms, gym bags, or travel kits, where the compact nature of bar soap proves to be practical and space-saving.

The affordability of bar soap is another significant factor in its enduring appeal. Generally, bar soap is less expensive compared to its liquid counterparts, making it an accessible option for a wide range of budgets. This cost-effectiveness, combined with its longevity, makes bar soap a practical choice for everyday use.

However, it's essential to acknowledge that bar soap does face some challenges. Hygiene concerns, particularly the possibility of bacteria accumulation on the bar, can deter some users. Nonetheless, proper storage and usage practices, such as allowing the bar to dry between uses and using a clean soap dish, can mitigate these concerns and ensure the soap remains hygienic.

In conclusion, bar soap's enduring appeal lies in its simplicity, environmental benefits, versatility, and affordability. While modern alternatives offer various advantages, bar soap continues to hold a special place in personal care routines. Its ability to adapt to contemporary needs while maintaining traditional values ensures that it remains a valuable choice for many. As consumers increasingly seek products that combine efficacy with environmental responsibility, bar soap stands out as a timeless and practical option in the realm of personal hygiene.

THE END